コロナ、わが友よ
Corona, our friend

マンフレッド・クラメス
Manfred Krames

この本の元はドイツ語版です。

私は 15 年間、日本に住んでいたので、

是非とも日本のみなさんに紹介したいと思い、

知り合いの石井さん（ヒカルランドの社長）に頼みました。

インターネットやメディアのコメントには、はっきり言ってうんざりです。

病状やロックダウン、あるいは経済的な影響についてばかりで、

誰一人として本当の原因を明らかにしません。

そこで、これらとは違う角度の必要性を感じました。

人の意識が変われば、どんな問題でも解決できます。

すべてが正しい理解から始まります。

ドイツから日本のみなさんの健康を祈っています。

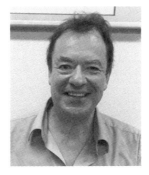

M. クラメス

CONTENTS

※「はじめに」「おわりに」の日本語は直訳ではなく、著者が日本人の心に合わせて書いた文章です。メッセージは翻訳、あるいは意訳です。

ブックデザイン　takaokadesign
編集　佐藤雅美

はじめに

　この世界に、悪いだけのものはありません。すなわち、CoVid-19パンデミックには良い面もあります。この物質主義の社会では、お金を稼ぐことやお金で買える"自由"が盲信され、誰も死や病気について考えようとしませんでした。どちらも生まれた瞬間から決まっていることなのに。そして、全世界がこのような悲惨な状況に陥っても、多くの人が、自分だけは平気という幻想を抱いています。

　コロナのおかげで、ようやく私たちは、地球上での限られた時間を認識することができました。これから先、新しい考え方や意識で、改めて生き続けられるでしょうか。それは、永遠に続くものは一つもないと知ること。そして、あの世に持っていけるものは一つもない。銀行口座の残高ではなく、他人や周りの環境、そして地球のことを、もっと真剣に考えるべきではないか、ということです。

　先進工業国の政府にとっては、経済成長がすべてです。

　そのために、仕事で厳しいノルマが課せられ、学生時代からすでに巨大なプレッシャーがかけられ、多くの人が苦しんで、元気さを失い、病気になっています。爆発的に増加している心の病が、その証拠の一つでしょう。特に敏感な人や直感に優れた人は、ずっと以前から、政治、社会、産業の何かがおかしいんじゃないかと感じていましたが、彼らも社会に適応するしかありませんでした。

　物質的な価値とお金に依存するあまり、人間が本来持っている愛情と同情が消えてしまったように見えます。そうした間違った価値観は、"人間の自然"に反発するものだからです。今起こっている全世界的なパラダイムシフトは、こうした精神的な苦しみからの帰結でしょう。天の知性（または神のような存在）が、苦しむ人たちの悲鳴を聞いて答えたのではないでしょうか。コロナが、その答えです。

　かつても、苦しむ魂の叫び声によって、天罰が下ったことがありました。

　1918年、毒ガスと大量の破壊兵器が使われ、数え切れないほどの人間が命を失った第一次世界大戦の終わり頃、

突然インフルエンザが発生して、世界中で 5 千万人もの死者が出ました。不思議なことに、このインフルエンザは、被害者の年齢が 20 歳から 40 歳の間に限られていました。もしかして、神のような存在が兵士の数を減らし、そして、これ以上、若い世代が召集されないように立てた作戦ではなかったでしょうか。

　母なる自然に対する残忍な乱獲、ひどい汚染、羊や牛のクローン開発など、私たちはいろいろな罪を犯しています。そして、消費者が安く肉を買うために、沢山のクジラとイルカが殺害され、毎日何千頭の牛や豚がひどい飼い方をされ、鶏がストレスで死んでしまうほど狭いかごに沢山詰め込まれています。それゆえ、自然が反撃を始めたのでしょう。もう、人間という"害虫"を駆除するしかないと。この天罰から学んで意識を変える人間が、何人残るでしょうか？

　外出禁止のために、久々に良い本を手に入れたり、家族とゲームを楽しんだりした人がいるようです。または、外

でお酒を飲む代わりに家族を思いやったり、外食の代わりに誰かと一緒に料理をした人もいるでしょう。混雑したクラブで踊るのではなく、家族や友人と電話で話した人もいるでしょう。必要のない消費や旅行で気晴らしする代わりに、将来や人生を真剣に考えることも、決して悪いことではありません。コロナのおかげで世の中が変わりつつあります。スマートフォンという「デジタル・パンデミック」が人類の健康に悪い影響を与え続けていますが、いずれ消えていくことでしょう。

　私が30年間学んできた最も古い医学、アーユルヴェーダの素晴らしい教えを一言でいうと：「自然の法（母なる自然および人間の内なる自然）に反する行いが、悪い結果を生む」。それは、不幸や病気、苦しみなど。単純にいえば、不自然なことが不健康のもとである、ということです。不自然な肥料、および電磁波（特にＧ５）、ワクチン、不自然に速い人生の速度など。

　コロナは今、社会的なパラダイムシフトを起こすところです。この警報が良い勉強となって、人間の意識が変わるでしょうか？　つまり、コロナの後（後があればですが）、

自然をより敬うでしょうか？　そして、他の生き物に対して愛情が生まれるでしょうか？　変なウイルス研究をやめられるでしょうか？　私にとって、このような問題は犠牲者の数よりも重要です。

　防護服、使い捨て手袋、マスクなどのほとんどが中国で製造されており、とんでもない依存を引き起こしました。抗生物質と多くの医療用製品も、おかげで不足しています。それがどれほど危険であるか、今のパンデミックが示してくれています。コロナよ、ありがとう。しかし、一体なぜ人権を踏みにじる国に工場を移したり、その国の製品を輸入しているのでしょうか？　それは、より安いものを求める消費者の需要に、業界が応えているからです。したがって、責任を感じない私たち消費者も非難されることになります。もしかして私たちの心にも、ウイルスのような悪玉が巣くってしまったのかもしれません。

　ウイルスというものは、環境に合わせて変異することを知っていましたか？　つまり、ウイルスは賢くなるという

ことです。一方、人間はどうでしょうか？　過去にあった多くの伝染病から、一体何を学んだでしょうか？　最終的に、何も変わってないではないですか？　つまり、ウイルスのほうが人間より賢いということです。少なくとも私たちは、自然に反することが危険だと知るべきでしょう。そして、変なクローン開発や遺伝子工学をやめるべきだったと思いませんか？　欲深さに切りがないから、結局、今、高い代償を払わなければなりません。

　25年ほど前に英国では、食肉用に処理された牛の骨を粉末にして、肉牛や乳牛に食わせていました。つまり、殺された「仲間」をエサにしたということです。その結果はBSE、つまり狂牛病という致死性神経病。この病気は、最終的に人間にもうつってしまいました。それは当たり前のことです。自然の暗示は、我々に届かなければならないのですから。

　数万羽のメンドリを窮屈な檻に入れておくと、その多くがストレスで死にます。それが鳥インフルエンザの原因の

一つであり、人間への復讐だろうという声が少なくありません。いまだに政府は、それを禁止する法律を成立させていません。産卵鶏として役に立たないひよこを生殺しにすることも許可されています。しかも、世界で毎月５千万回以上も。

　コロナの話に戻りましょう。イタリアで死亡率が特に高い原因の一つは、抗生物質の店頭販売が原因だと言われています。処方箋は必要ないので、ちょっとした病気ですぐ抗生物質を飲むのが習慣になっています。したがって、今一番、抗生物質が必要なときに効かなくなってしまいました。日本はどうですか？　ちょっとした風邪で医者がすぐに抗生物質を出すので、同じではないでしょうか？　それだけではなく、牛や豚が残酷な飼育法でも病気にならないために、エサに沢山の抗生物質が混ぜられています。それもまた、私たちの体に入ってきます。したがって、人間はコロナを発生させただけでなく、もともと私たちに備わっている大事な免疫系も駄目にしました。サッカーであれば、それを「二重オウンゴール」と呼ぶでしょう。こんな馬鹿

なことが、宇宙の中にあるだろうか⁉

　しかしながら、政治と産業に罪を着せるだけでは解決になりません。我々、安い肉を買う消費者にも責任がないとは言えません。動物のために菜食主義を考えるのもよいことでしょう。また、生物兵器として危険なウイルスを生産する国をボイコットするために、その国の製品を一切買わない方法もあります。

　デジタル技術とインターネットのおかげで、世界はガラス張りになりました。不都合な科学者の意見を永遠に隠すことができない時代です。つまり、私たち消費者には、それを買わないという偉大な権力が与えられているのです。私たちが意識していないだけです。そのために、ソーシャルネットワークを利用することを考えてください。

　デジタルネットワークを賢く利用するのは、今のところ、Greta Thunberg（グレタ・トゥーンベリ）だけのようです。彼女は確かにナイーブな部分がありますが、一生懸命、全世界の人の目を覚ます活動を行っています。なんて素晴

らしいことでしょう！　私たちはみんな若い頃に、理想的な考えと夢を持っていたではないですか！　社会人になるにつれ残念ながら、その理想主義が単なる消費主義に変わってしまいました。しかし、今の若い世代の夢を絶対、破ってはいけません。

　どこかの無責任な一人が間違いを起こすと全世界に影響があることを、我々に痛いほど教えてくれたのは、コロナウイルスです。今こそ、この課題と解決法を腑に落とさないと、次のパンデミックでは絶対生き残れないでしょう。

　ここで、医療および看護専門職の人々、公共サービスや供給業の人々、電車やバスの運転手、スーパーで働く人々、記者、インターネットのプロバイダー、農家、食品メーカーの人々に、感謝の言葉を残したいと思います。彼らの勇気ある活動を見習いましょう。

　あなたの周りには、家を出るのを恐れている老人や病気の人がいるに違いありません。その人たちに買い物やその他の支援を提供できます。玄関先にバッグを置くことができます。両親や子どもたちが遠くに住んでいるなら、健康

について尋ねましょう。彼らの恐れを取り除きましょう。勇気と希望を与え、必要なところを助けて、狂った買い物客は無視しましょう！

　もし"向こう岸"に行く時が来たら、私たちは一銭も持って行けません。人生の名声や権力も、あの世では役に立ちません。善事、つまり他人にしてあげたことしか価値がないのです。その道を歩むために、恐れがあなたを征服することを許さないでください。その道のために必要な道具が、愛と勇気です。

マンフレッド・クラメス

Foreword

This book is not meant to be flown over or read in a fast forward mode. Take your time, sit down comfortably, put a cup of tea aside, turn off all noise making devices, then allow the texts and pictures to speak to you. It is not the book's intention to influence you, or to push your opinion into a certain direction. It is perfectly alright to come to different conclusions.

In any case, the epic scale of the present pandemic is of such over-whelming dimension, that it demands a perspective different from the mainstream media altogether. In the wake of generalizing the situation, or focusing on daily difficulties and restrictions, we risk losing sight of the meaning of this catastrophe along with its root cause.

The entire world is lamenting on the nonsense of tough lock downs, and that our life is not the same any more. For this, a tiny little virus is blamed, enlarged to a horrifying super size, as displayed on background images on almost every TV news show. Internet contributions focus on "manipulated death toll", "false information", "nonsense of counter measurements" and the like, in addition to the many conspiracy theories, while, in doing so, the quest for finding the origin of this "social pathogenesis" falls under the table. China has become the scapegoat, but that too is much too easy, I feel.

In Germany, millions of people anxiously await the day hair dressers reopen, or wonder when they can go to parties again. With our minds occupied with such silly little matters, we run danger to not learn from this event. If we do not learn our lesson from this pandemic, it would have occurred in vain, which subsequently might trigger yet another catastrophe. From the viewpoint of cosmic intelligence, or god, if you are religious, every plague, every natural disaster carries a message. Nothing happens by chance.

Most naturopaths and open-minded doctors around the world recognize a suffering psyche behind many physical illnesses, and their number is growing fast. "Inconformity as a sign from our soul" or "Disease as message from our body" and the like titles are to be found in every book store in Germany, supported by the masses and the media. However, with our sickening planet, a living organism it is after all, it is not different. Just like a stroke is a wake up call for the patient, this pandemic is a stress signal from Mother Earth, from Mother Nature.

If we ignore her warning sign, if we not take her message serious now, if being concerned about money and pleasure is all we are concerned about, another catastrophe might follow. Looking at the selfish reaction of some profit oriented business owners these days, and how many try to take advantage of the situation, I am pretty certain that this will be the scenario in due time. Politicians, too, use the crisis as a stepladder to advance their career, pretending that all their actions are for the better of their beloved citizens.

In most countries one can observe a decline of morals and ethic values over the past decades. In fact, one could speak of an unparalleled paradigm shift in human history, in which consumerism, capitalism and greed for money and power is all that matters. Amidst this dense materialistic environment and mental suffering, corona appears, paralyzing the entire global economy with one single strike. This is so shockingly "effective" that most people do not even realize what's going on. Whatever can be done to avoid another epidemic should be done. Those sitting around doing nothing but lamenting are a sub-cause of the outbreak. We all have opportunities to actively add something to improve the situation. Let's use them. Putting all our hopes on a vaccine is the wrong way. This might, as with any human conformity, ease the symptoms somewhat, but won't get to the root cause, disabling lasting recovery.

Once you finish the picture part, lay the book aside and contemplate a bit on the impressions, allowing them to reach your consciousness. In the chapter following we shall go more into the depths. The insights have neither to do with a certain worldview or esoteric, nor with any religious aspects. If I accomplish to elevate the awareness of some intelligent, open minded people, the book was worth while the effort.

May 1st 2020

Manfred Krames

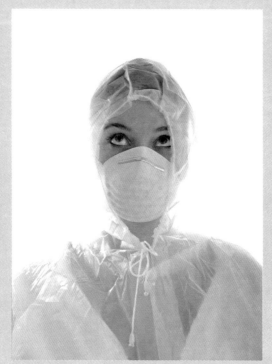
Clarissa Schwarz/ pixelio.de

自己中心的な冷たい社会で、
人と人の距離がさらに遠くなることに、
心が痛みます。

In a cold hearted elbow society a
ban on social contacting causes more
mental torment than elsewhere.

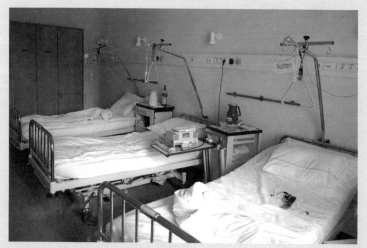

by-sassi/ pixelio.de

死んだ3人はすでに埋葬されました。
次のコロナ犠牲者に
ベッドが必要だから。

The three dead ones had been buried
at once, as their beds are needed
by the next corona victims.

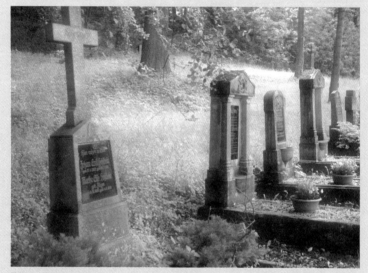
Webwebwebber/ pixelio.de

私たちのただひとつの真の贅沢は
生きる時間があることです。
コロナがそれを意識させてくれました。

The only true luxury we
have is TIME. Corona
made us aware of it.

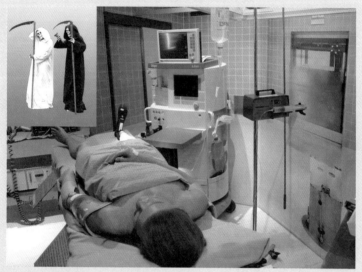

Dieter Schütz / pixelio.de

こんなに大勢が苦しんでいる。
これほどひどい目に遭うなんて、
人間は一体何を間違えましたか?

So much suffering. How could it
have come this far? What
have we done wrong?

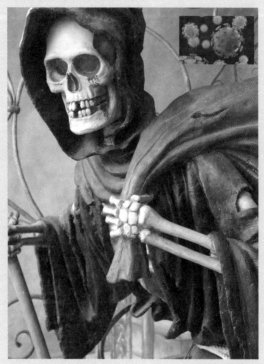

コロナは突然変異しましたが、
似たウイルスが以前にもありました。

The mutation of the corona virus is
a new one, but similar viruses
did exist previously.

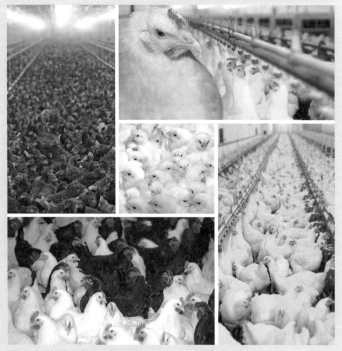

たとえば、メンドリ何万匹を
狭いかごに押し込んで
ひどい飼い方をする国で。
結果として、鶏が大量に病気にかかって、
ストレスで死んでしまいました。
鳥インフルエンザの発生。

For instance in places where chicken
had so little space that they grew
sick or died of stress. The
bird flu evolved.

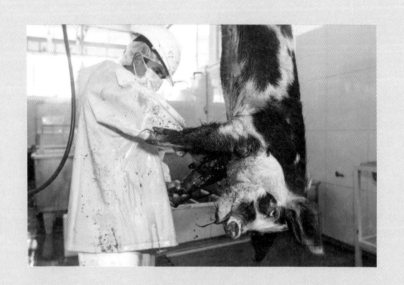

豚たちこそ人間にちゃんと扱われていません。
それは養豚場だけでなく、
食肉処理場こそ残酷。

Pigs are not treated in a permissable
way either. In regards to farming
as well as slaughtering.

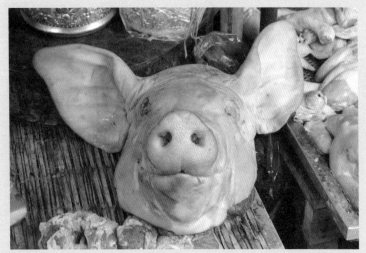

Igor Sokolov/ 123RF

結果として、豚インフルエンザが
人間への警報か…?

Does Mother Nature take revenge
for what we cause to her?
The swine flu as a signal?

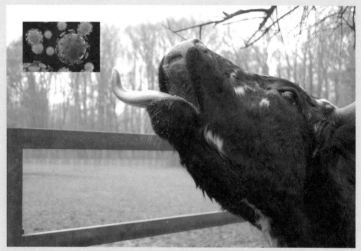

INQ/ pixelio.de
Christian Daum/ pixelio.de

食肉処理された牛の骨を粉末にし、それを
エサに混ぜ、生きている牛に与えました。
つまり"仲間"を食べさせた。
すると神経がおかしくなって、
BSE（狂牛病）が発生し、
結局、人間にもうつりました。当然です。
我々にメッセージが届かなければ
意味がないのだから……。

When cattle was fed with pulverized
bones from their slaughtered "friends"
BSE broke out, a deadly nervous
disease that killed men too.

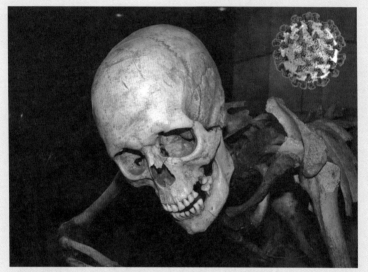

Dieter Schütz/ pixelio.de

コロナの発生について、
様々な理論があります。
ひとつは、ある国の研究室から、
生物兵器のために作った
危ないウイルスが流出した。
つまり、このパンデミックを起こしたのは、
人間です。

There are several theories on the
genesis of corona. One is a leaking
virus from a Chinese laboratory for
biological weapons. Fact remains
that man has has wronged nature.

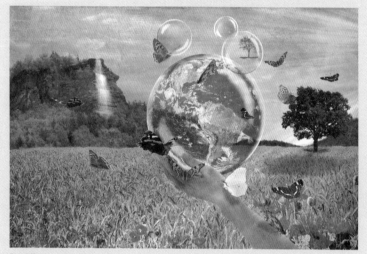

Bernd Kasper/ pixelio.de

素晴らしい大自然が、コロナウイルスで
伝えたい暗示とは、一体何？
それとも、我々人間は
減らさなければいけない "害虫"
になったのでしょうか？

Our beautiful earth. What she
tries to convey through corona?
Or is it just a decimation
of the human pests?

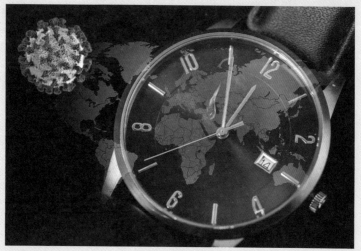

Bernd Kasper/ pixelio.de

人類が滅亡した後、母なる地球は
やっと回復できるでしょう。
しかし、生き残った人々は
同じ失敗を繰り返すでしょうか？

After mankind has been decimated,
Mother Earth can breathe a sigh of
relief. Will the survivors relearn?

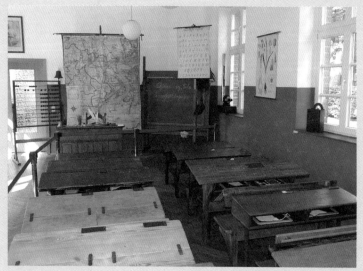

Dieter Schütz/ pixelio.de

多くの子どもたちの頭に、
本の知識やデータが詰め込まれました。
同時に彼らの心を育て、
意識と責任感を伸ばしたならば、
こんな状態にならなかったでしょう。

The heads of many had been crammed
with book knowledge, facts and data.
Had we cultivated their hearts as well,
it would not have gotten that far.

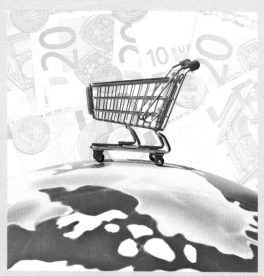

Thorsten Wengert/ pixelio.de

しかし、そういった価値観が、
産業国ではあまり伝わっていません。
金儲けと経済力が第一。

Spiritual values like ethics, collective re-
sponsibility and self-realization
do not count in the West. In the
end it's all about money.

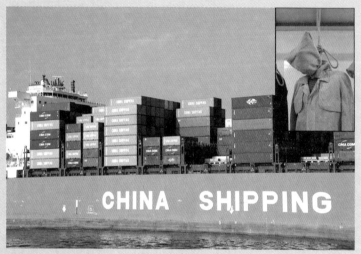

Bernd Sterzl/ pixelio.de

抗生物質、防護マスク、防護服などの
医療品を、
人権を無視する国で安く作らせています。
たとえ、その国に依存しても。
利益のためなら、我々人間は何でもする。

Antibiotics, protective masks and suits
etc. we let manufacture in countries
that disrespect human rights, even if
that causes a risky dependence. Why?

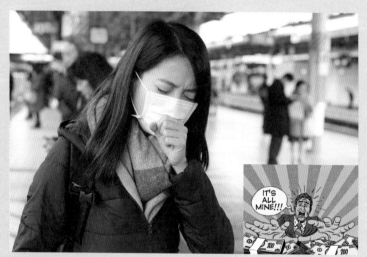

Thorsten Wengert/ pixelio.de

通勤できなくなると、
大量の失業者が生まれるでしょう。
コロナで大儲けしようとした
企業の大物たちよ、
地獄に落ちればよい。

If commuting to work gets worse,

lots of people will end in poverty.

May those trying to make a fortune

on Corona go to hell.

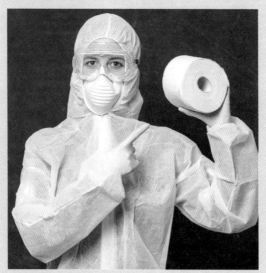

Massonforstock/ 123RF

ある消費者がトイレットペーパーを
50 個も買い込んだ。
1個がひと月もつにも関わらず。
自己中心の最悪の表現。

ところで、インド人は、
お尻を水と石鹸で洗います。
そのほうが衛生的。試してみませんか?

Egoists shopped 50 rolls of toilet paper,
in spite of 1 roll lasting over a month.

By the way, Japanese toilets have a built-in shower
instead using paper. And in India, people wash their butt
with water and soap, which is much more hygienic.

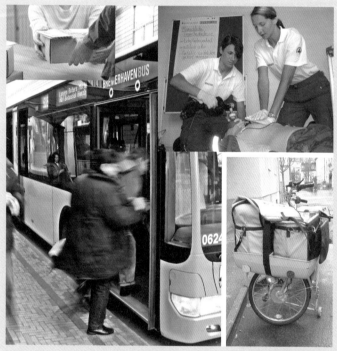

Paket / 123RF
Enysipel / pixelio.de
Andrea Kusajda / pixelio.de
Kunstart.net / pixelio.de

こんなとき感謝しなければいけないのは、
スーパーで働く人、電車やバスの運転手、
配送業者、エネルギー供給業の人々、
そして特に、医療関係者です。
コロナが彼らを英雄にする。

Gratitude to all cashiers, bus and taxi drivers, deliverers, electricity suppliers
and those in medical professions.
Corona turned you into heroes.

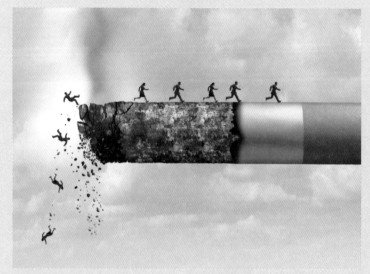

Lightwise / 123RF

いくらお金があっても、
国民の健康がなければ、経済は破綻します。
これからは、免疫系を強化して、
不健康な習慣をやめなければ。

Nothing matters more than health. The
entire economy is down and devastated if
we are not well. Let us strengthen our
immune system, and give up bad habits!

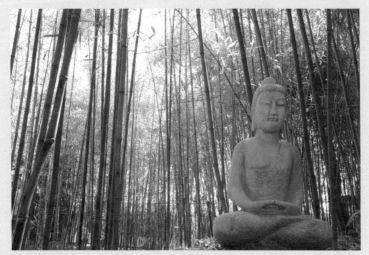

Thorsten Scholl/ pixelio.de

「もし、世界中の木がすべて筆であって、
海がすべて墨であっても、
人類の苦しみを描くには足りません」
釈迦

"If all trees in the world were pens, and all
oceans ink, not would it be enough to de-
scribe the suffering on earth."
Buddha

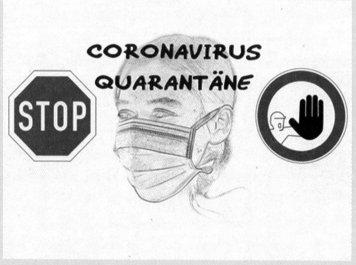

Thommy Weiss/ pixelio.de

以前にもウイルスが発生し、
変異しながら耐性を獲得した。
人間は変わらずに、昔の失敗を繰り返した。
つまり、ウイルスより愚か！

Humans have not really learned their
lesson yet, but viruses did. They mutated
and became resistant. How smart!

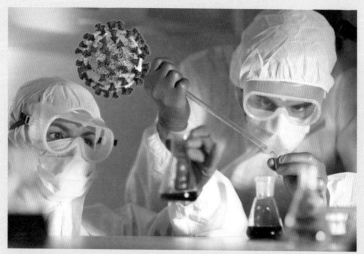

dolgachov / 123RF

もし、科学が生物兵器の研究に
悪用されるならば、
その危険なウイルスが流出するならば、
我々みんなにも責任がある。
なぜなら、それに反対しなかったから。

If science is misused to breed biological
weapons from viruses, we all are to be
blamed if those are used, or escape by mi-
stake. We failed to prevent it.

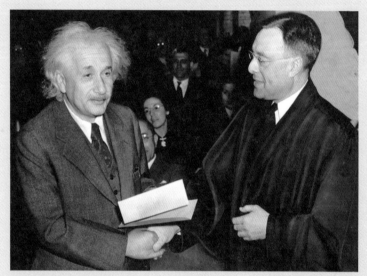

Einstein erhält 1940 die amerikanische Einbürgerungsurkunde

「人間の愚かさと宇宙の広さは、
両方とも無限である。
しかし後者には、まだ疑問の余地がある」
アルバート・アインシュタイン

"The stupidity of men, and the vastness of
space, both are infinite. But I'm not quite
sure about the latter."
Albert Einstein

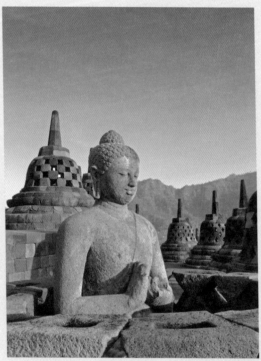

Dr. Stephan Barth/ pixelio.de

「どの病気にも良い薬があるが、
無知にはない」
釈迦

"There is a medicine for all illnesses,
except for ignorance."
Buddha

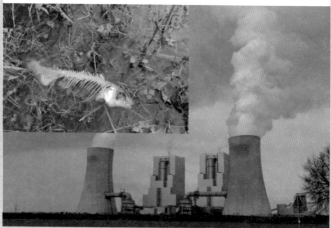

Alexander Hauk / pixelio.de
M. Großmann / pixelio.de
Frank Gronendahl / pixelio.de

科学者たちが今、発見したのは、
二酸化炭素濃度とコロナの関係。
すなわち、公害のひどいところに
感染者が多い。
日光が当たらないと免疫系が弱まる。
環境をより真剣に考える理由になればよい。

Scientists discovered a connection
between Co2-levels and a CoVid19
proneness, respectively a weakened
immune systeme. A good reason to take
environmental pollution and health
more serious in the future.

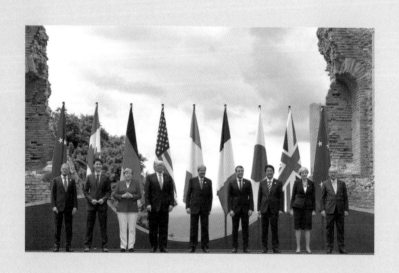

多大な犠牲とともに、人類は
このパンデミックを乗り越えるでしょう。
ただし、何も変わらなければ、
次のパンデミックが我々を全滅させる。

それを防ぐために、科学者はいらない。
頭のいい奴らより、
叡智のある指導者が必要。
そして、真の価値観を伝える教育と。

With great losses, we'll survive. But if
we not change, the next pandemic
will wipe us all out for sure.

For this, we not need academics, as "clever minds"
caused the problem in the first place, but wise leaders
and an education system conveying different values.

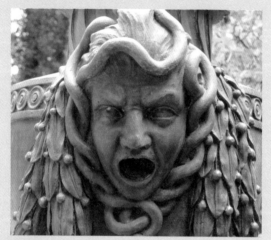

Ralf Meilen/ pixelio.de

人類の歴史の中で
人間が起こした残酷な苦しみは
他の生き物より、はるかに多い。
闘わなければいけないのはウイルスではなく、
「無責任」と「欲」。

The physical and mental torment we
inflict to each other is immeasurable.
It is not viruses that need to be
tackled, but greed and selfishness.

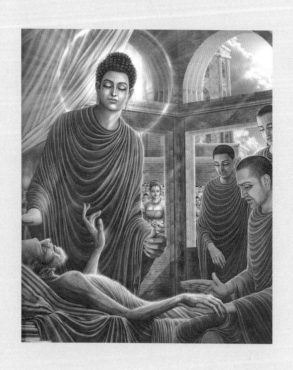

危険に直面した時に他人を助ける人こそ、
真の英雄だ。
それに比べて、征服者は
ただのウジ虫である。

The one who helps others in the face of
danger, is a hero indeed, a true Christian.
Compared to him, the great conquerors
are meaningless worms.

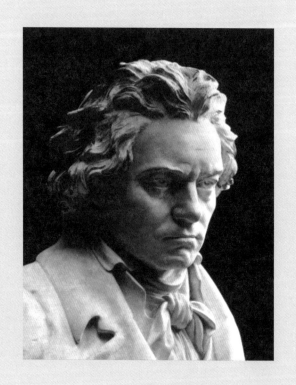

「あなたの人生をより幸せにするのは
愛しかできません。愛こそすべて」
ルートヴィヒ・ヴァン・ベートーベン

"Love, and love alone, can make your life
happier."
Ludwig van Beethoven

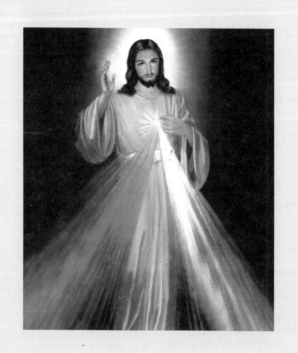

悪魔や恐怖に惑わされないで！
愛と信頼で生きよう。

Do not be misled, neither by Satan
nor by fear! Live by love and
trust.

日本のみなさんへの
ボーナス

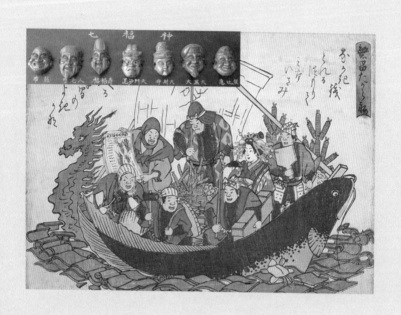

ある友人が言った。
「災いは神様からの恋文だ」
20年後、僕はその意味がやっと分かった。
災いがなかったら、我々人間は
何一つ変わらないでいたでしょう。

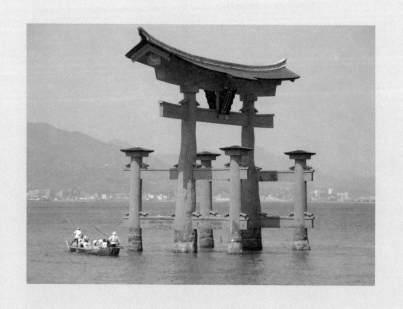

時々思う。
日本の神々がまだいるとしたら、
きっと失望しているに違いない。
日本人よ、
なぜ日本人の細胞に反する
西洋化に走るのか。
元々の素晴らしい文化と叡智に
戻ったらいいではないか。

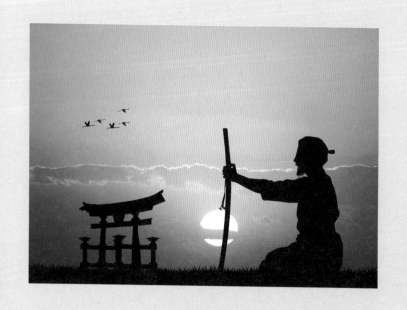

何を信じていいか、
誰を信用していいか分からないときは、
感覚に任すしかない。
直感が、道筋を示してくれる。
勘が、矢を的の中心へと導く。

それこそ武士道の奥義である。

おわりに

　コロナが蔓延している国々の中で、死亡率が一番低いのはドイツです。死亡率が高いイタリアと違って、抗生物質は医師によって処方されなければなりません。つまり、深刻な病気にのみ使われます。しかし、必要があっても、多くの医師はできるだけ抗生物質を避けようとします。なぜならば、抗生物質は体内に耐性をつくるので、ここぞという時に効かなくなるからです。

　日本はドイツと同じように、抗生物質の使用には医師の処方が必要です。しかし、かなり軽い風邪のような症状でも、それが処方されるのが普通のやり方です。おかげで体が慣れてしまって、もう効果があまりありません。

　より体に優しく、もっと自然な治療法への要望が、日本でも非常に大きくなりました。つまり東洋医学をより提供してほしいという声が、かつてないほど大きくなっています。しかし、政治家は依然、製薬に基づく西洋医学を守っています。たとえ多くの副作用があっても。それで一番喜

ぶのは製薬会社でしょう。彼らは売り上げが爆発的に増加したのですから。

　みなさんご存知の通り、日本の政治にとって、経済が第一です。もちろん経済成長は必要ですが、国民の健康が悪化するとどうなるか、コロナウイルスが痛いほど示してきました。ありがとう、コロナ。国民の健康（精神的な面も含めて）に問題があれば、経済は破綻し、何も意味がありません。

　しかし、それだけではありません。抗生物質は畜産にも使用されています。成長ホルモンや抗ストレスホルモンとともに。これらすべてが私たちの体内に入り込み、免疫システムを弱めます。安い肉をショッピングカートに追加するときは、是非、このことを覚えておいてください。

　環境に一切かまわずに、二酸化炭素を排出する国が、間接的にそうでない国の人々の免疫系を弱めているのは事実です。さらに、他国が発生させたPM2.5の雲が、日本に流れてくるケースも少なくありません。今こそ、コロナウイルスに感染しない方法は、強い免疫システムしかあり

ません。ですから、そういう環境を汚したり、人権を無視したりする国のモノを買い求めることで応援しないほうがいいと思いませんか？　商社は利益しか追求しないし、政治家はどこまで信用できるかわかりません。私たち消費者が持っている権限を、思いきり利用する方法を見逃さないでください。

　たとえ少し高くても、まともな国の製品を選びましょう。そして、肉のタンパク質の代わりに豆腐や玄米を食べれば、その食習慣に慣れている日本人の細胞は、きっと喜びます。そのほうが、自然にも健康にも最適です。さらに、これから気をつけてほしいのは、農薬が使われている農産物。これも、いろいろな病気を発生させ、免疫系を弱める原因になります。新型コロナウイルスからは何とか生き残るかもしれませんが、今こそ意識が変わらず、何も変更しないなら、次のパンデミックが絶対に最後だと思ってください。罪のない子どもたちが一番かわいそうです。結局、良くない製品や農産物を輸入するより、無農薬の国産を選択するほうが、みんなのためではないでしょうか？

　そうすると、昔から日本人に一番合う食習慣、および生活に戻れるかもしれません。おかげで、私たちがやっと自分らしく、あるいは日本人らしく生きることができるでしょう。もしそうなったら、コロナウイルスは、それほど悪いものではありません。

　すでに、良い影響が出てきています。酒場が閉まっているなら、早く家に帰って家族と一緒に過ごすサラリーマンたちの姿が見られます。企業の社長たちが在宅勤務に抵抗してできないと言ったのに、やってみれば、悪い結果は一つもありません。コロナのおかげで、良い実践ができました。こうした経験を重ねていって、パンデミックが収まった後も続けていけば、最高だと思いませんか？　日本のひどい通勤ラッシュが２割だけでも減れば十分です。

　もしかして、苦しんでいるワーカホリックを救うために、神のような存在が今の状態を起こしたかもしれません。つまり、日本人に必要な社会的な改革をプッシュしてくれたのであれば、ありがたいこと。そうした面から見れば、将来は決して暗くありません。しかし、今こそ意識が変わらなければ、せっかくのチャンスを見逃すことになってしま

います。何と、もったいないことでしょう。

　みなさん是非良い方向を向いて、メディアが送るひどいニュースばかりを見続けないでください。それこそ、免疫系を弱める原因となります。代わりに、久しぶりに家族で楽しいゲームをしたり、料理をしたり、誰かと散歩に行ったりしてはいかがでしょうか？　そして、子どもたちに本を読んであげたり、時間を一緒に過ごしたりしましょう。人間関係を深くする大きなチャンスに違いありません。

Epilogue

Nothing in this world is totally negative. And so the CoVid-19 pandemic too, has a positive side. In our materialistic society, blinded by consumerism and pseudo-freedom, we have all supplanted the uncomfortable thought of death and illness, although both are inevidable since birth. May the whole world fall into misery, it will not affect me, so the illusion of many. Thanks to Corona, we have been made aware of our limited time on earth, which hopefully will enable us to restart with a new awareness.

Economic growth is a priority for governments in most industrialized countries. As a result, tough requirements in the job world, as well as a tremendous pressure that starts already at school, all of which is mirrored in the sharp increase of psychosomatic disorders in those countries. The farsighted and sensitive among us in particular have long felt that something is wrong with politics, society and industry, but have to adapt to survive. The addiction to prosperity has almost completely erased the humane, the loving and compassionate, the considerate in us. In my opinion, this global shift in values, which adolescents much suffering, must have triggered a mental torment that may have been heard by a higher power, or a divine intelligence. The reply: Corona.

For once the screaming of lost souls was so loud that it was answered: in 1918, near the end of World War I, where poisonous gases and other means of mass destruction was used, killing millions in a most horrible way, all of a sudden a flu broke out, resulting into 50 Million deaths worldwide. Unlike usual, just 20 to 40 year olds were affected. Could perhaps a higher power have tried to eliminate soldiers and preventing further drafting in by order?

Brutal exploitation of mother earth, cloning of sheep and goats, cruel killing of many whales and dolphins, animal testing for drugs, the grotesque and painful slaughter of thousands of cattle, pigs and chickens every day, so that we can buy cheap meat, as well as the global pollution of sky, water and earth may have left nature with no choice but to take a counter-strike against humanity, as a pest control, so to say. Let us see whether this act will bear fruit, whether people will change afterwards.

Thanks to curfew, some have picked up a good book after a long time or played board games with the family. Family domesticity instead of absence. Thoughtfulness instead of rumbling in a pub. Cooking together instead of dining out. Talking on the phone with family and friends instead of dancing in a crowded club. Thinking about the future and life instead of distractions from unnecessary consumerism and long-distance travel. Smartphones and i-phones, our "digital pandemic", still distract from the essentials of life, but that will change too, some day. Generally speaking, Corona has triggered a reflection within some of us. If there is an "after", will we act in a more meaningful, respectful, loving, helpful and grateful manner, or will we fall back into the old patterns? As for me, this question is more vital than the death count of victims.

Protective suits, disposable gloves and masks, almost all are made in Asia, along with antibiotics and other medical components. But why, I ask myself, are we moving factories to countries that trample on our values and on human rights?

Because avarice is "cool" and because the industry supplies to our demand for cheapness. So we, the consumers, are partially to be blamed.

Viruses are known to mutate, which means they evelove intelligently. And man? Have we developed and learned from the many epidemics and pandemics in the past? Shouldn't we have known that acting against nature is dangerous? Whether this is cloning, genetic engineering or virus breeding, we played with fire and now must pay a high price.

Ayurveda, the world's most ancient medical system, studied by me for 30 years, basically says this: To any action against nature (outer nature and humans' internal nature) follows a negative consequence in the form of sickness, unhappiness or suffering. To put it more banal: Anything unnatural is unhealthy. If we teach only this to our children, it will elevate the consciousness of generations by manifold.

For decades scientists are warning of the harmful effects from electro-magnetic waves as radiating from cellular phones, WiFi-routers and the like, and that it weakens the body's immune system. Unnaturally high waves in the micro and giga periphery are surrounding us all day long. But G5 technology will surpass those harmful effects manifold.

When Dr. Rashid Buttar found a connection between G5 exposure and proneness to corona infection, his YouTube contribution got deleted within a few days. Perhaps he should not have mentioned Bill Gates, who is also an investor in the research of corona viruses.

Vandana Shiva, an Indian nuclear scientist and environmentalist, further found out that Bill Gates cooperates with Monsanto (infamous for the production of Glycosat), in an attempt to digitalize the patenting of gene manipulated seeds . . . and viruses. Her sites had been deleted, too. However, such news only lead us astray to get into conspiracy theories, of which I am an opponent.

Even if I could proof the involvement of industrial giants in the USA and their research funding in Wuhan, China, what good would it do? We cannot undo the damage done. Fact remains that men have wronged nature. Shouldn't we have known better? Shouldn't we all have realized that messing with nature is a dangerous game? Whether it is gene manipulation, cloning, virus breeding or the employment of electro magnetic radiation, strong enough to boil our cells.

25 years ago, a certain European country had ground the bones of slaughtered cows into powder, feeding it to live cattle and dairy cows who, as a matter of fact, thus ate their own relatives. The result: BSE, or mad cow disease, a fatal nerve disease that swapped over to humans. Well, somehow the message had to get through.

Keeping tens of thousands of chickens in cramped cages, many of which died of stress, was one of the causes of the bird flu, taking revenge on humans. To date, our governments have not passed laws to ban this practise. Slaughtering live chicks that are useless as egg-laying chickens is also permitted. It happens thousand times hourly around the globe.

Back to Corona, our friend. Why the death rate is particularly high in Italy may be due to prescription-free over-the-counter sales of antibiotics, taken there as self-treatment for every (mostly harmless) infections or flues. The body thus built up resistance over time, so that now, when antibiotics are vital, they lost their effectiveness. Antibiotics in the feed of pigs, chickens and cows, to prevent them from getting sick and surviving the stress, ends up on our plate, too. So man not only triggered Corona, he also disabled his immune system. In football we would call that a "double own goal".

But let's not just blame politics and industry. Everyone who shops cheap meat is partly responsible for the miserable factory farming and cruel slaughter. Anyone who buys imported goods from countries producing biological weapons or despising human rights, is complicit! The only thing that has developed over the past 5000 years seems to be technology. If only it would have been used for a revolution than for distraction and amusement. How easy it would be to boycott such countries via social networks, preventing their products from being bought. We have to hit them where it causes pain: money, profit, economical success. We, the customers and consumers, have the power, but are unaware of it.

Thanks to digital technology and the Internet, the world has become a glass house. Certain countries can no longer silence inconvenient researchers or academics or millionaires, making them disappear without anyone exposing it ONLINE. But what do we do with the available information? We get upset and remain passive. Greta Thunberg is an exception. She feels the suffering of our planet and tries to mobilize and sensitize the whole world. How great! Such idealism, which we all had as youths, must not be taken away from us! Corona, a mutant intelligent virus, now shows us the consequences of passiveness.

Our buying behavior, our travel destinations, our investments in other countries etc. are all an effective means of pressure, as long as we are honest to ourselves, instead getting corrupt.

Ultimately, we are being tested now, on a small or big scale. Are we selfish, or do we bravely stand up for our fellow human beings in need? Corona is our friend! Do not be afraid! Fear is the actual enemy. Fear triggers wrong decisions and subsequently paralyzes our immune system, which we desperately need now. Let us take an example of the people in medical and nursing professions, those in public service, suppliers, taxi and bus drivers, cashiers, reporters, electricity and internet providers, farmers and food suppliers. Shouldn't we all give them a helping hand now?

I am sure there are old or sick ones near you, afraid to leave the house. You could offer them shopping or any other assistance. Bags can be put in front of their door. (Same with the procurement of medicines for those in quarantine.) Let's be concerned about our parents and children if they live far away, giving them a call, especially if we have lost contact over a prolonged period. Corona offers us a chance to reconnect and to heal wounds. Let's reduce fear of the scared ones. Let's give courage, hope and help where it is needed and let us disregard the crazy shoppers and scarers! In doing so, Corona could become our friend.

Thanks to this tiny little virus, we begin to realize that life is not eternal, that we are vulnerable, fragile and subject to death. Being unaware of our short life span and limited recourses is what caused the problem in the first place. In fact, infinite exploitation of a finite planet is nothing but suicide. We had been mislead by false illusions all along the path, while billionaires fight an invisible war on earth that is all about power, no matter what. Not the disease should be blamed, but that what caused it. Not the little virus should be fought, but ignorance and irresponsibility. Corona has become the scapegoat for a phenomena that is nothing but a cancerous form of capitalism.

When we leave this world, we cannot take a single penny with us. Nobody can accompany us. Any achievement or fame won't be useful. The only thing we can take along is the good we did to others. Our deeds matter, nothing else. This is the essence of all religions. Therefore, do not allow fear to conquer you, but love and courage. Do not trust smart logic or academic talk by scientists, but instead listen to your inner voice. Trust your gut feeling, your intuition and 6th sense, or however you may call it. Awareness alone can transform us, can turn us into better human beings. Do not allow others to entice you! Weakness triggered by fear is the first step, so watch out!

Manfred Krames

マンフレッド・クラメス
（Prof. h. c. Manfred Krames）

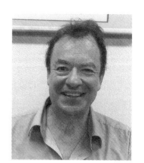

・1963 年、ドイツ最古の都市
　Trier（トリーア）で生まれる
・20 歳まで学校教育（経済学短期大学）
・日本で 2 年以上、仏教の勉強（福井県）
・東京で 3 年間、中国伝統医学の勉強
・日本アーユルヴェーダ研究会のメンバーに（主宰：幡井勉教授）
・Dr. U. K. クリシュナ（グジャラートアーユルヴェーダ大学）と研究
・日本に住んで 11 年後 スリランカに移り、Dr. Upali Pilapitiya（政府のアー
　ユルヴェーダ研究センター）と他の専門家と 2 年、研究
・12 人のスタッフと Kandy（スリランカ）でアーユルヴェーダクリニックを開設
・スリランカのオープン国際大学で「アーユルヴェーダ教授」として名誉学位
　を取得

教育講師経験

・1997 年、ドイツのバーデンバーデン市で大アーユルヴェーダクリニックを開業
・1999 年、ドイツアーユルヴェーダ・アカデミーを開校、500 人以上の医療専
　門家に講義（その間ドイツの私立学校で一年間心理カウンセリングを勉強）
・2000−2005 年、ドイツ、ラトビア、イタリア、カナダ、日本、スリランカ、
　タイ、インドの大学で公共のスピーチ、講演会、セミナー etc.

・2006-2012 年、スリランカのタイ大使の提案によりタイでアーユルヴェーダを紹介。大学やロータリークラブなどで講義
・2013 年、いくつかの医療機関や総合的な診療のためのコンサルタント
・2015 年、日本へ戻り、心理カウンセリングとセミナー講師を務める

出版物:

・アーユルヴェーダに関する 5 冊の書籍をドイツの URANIA 社などで出版
・英語版のアーユルヴェーダ本をイギリスとアメリカで 4 冊出版
・仏教について 3 冊をバンコクとドイツで出版
・アジアの西洋化についての重要な書籍を 3 冊出版
・ドイツの医学雑誌や科学雑誌に多くの記事を執筆
・心身症の原因に関する本をドイツ医学専用出版社と日本で出版

メンバーシップ:
・日本ホリスティック医学協会、東京
・ドイツ心理カウンセラーの連盟協会 (VFP)
・国際医療ジャーナリスト協会
・アーユルヴェーダ保全社会、スリランカ

HP:https://mpk-japan.jimdofree.com/
(カウンセリングのお問い合わせもこちらへどうぞ)

Prof. h. c. Manfred Krames

Academic background in brief

Born 1963 in Germany

College for Economy (Tanki daigaku)

Study of Buddhism in Fukui-Ken, Japan (2 years)

Study of Shiatsu and Moxa at private academy in Tokyo

Member of the Japan Ayurveda Research Association under Prof. Ben Hatai

Study of Ayurveda with Dr. U. K. Krishna (Gujarat Ayurved University) as private tutor

Study of Ayurveda with Dr. Upali Pilapitiya (Director of the governmental Ayurveda Research Institute of Sri Lanka), later with Dr. M. Pushpa, Colombo

Eight visits to India, meeting various experts on Ayurveda

Further studies of traditional Chinese Medicine under Prof. Xiu University

Honorary degree of Professor from the Open International University, Sri Lanka

Teaching experience

Lectures in Japan on Ayurveda and Holistic Medicine in 1993 and 1994

Organizer and chief speaker of Ayurveda Seminar in Yokohama 1993

Regular lectures at the Open International University of Sri Lanka 1995

Speeches at various institutions in India, incl. Gujarat University 1996-98

Opening of Academy in Germany, 1999 - 2004, lecturing to over 300 medical professionals.

Public speeches at hospitals, clinics and institutions in Germany, Latvia,

Switzerland, Canada and Italy

Lectures at Bangkok Buddhist University and Rotary Clubs in Thailand

Chief guest speaker at the 2010 conference of the International Ayurveda Society, Pune, India

Publications

8 books on Ayurveda, published by various German publishers

3 books on psychosomatic disorders, published in England & USA

3 books on the changes of Thai society, published in Bangkok in Thai

1 documentary film on the misconceptions of westernized Ayurveda

10 lengthy articles for German psychological magazines and medical journals

Membership

Member of the Japan Holistic Medical Association

Member of the German Union of Medical Journalists

Member: Alternative Medicine Association of Germany

VFP, German Association for psychological counselors

コロナ、わが友よ：Corona, our friend

第一刷 2020年7月31日

著者 マンフレッド・クラメス

発行人 石井健資
発行所 株式会社ヒカルランド

〒162-0821 東京都新宿区津久戸町3-11 TH1ビル6F
電話 03-6265-0852 ファックス 03-6265-0853
http://www.hikaruland.co.jp info@hikaruland.co.jp

振替 00180-8-496587
本文・カバー・製本 中央精版印刷株式会社
DTP 株式会社キャップス
編集担当 TakeCO

コロナウイルスで気が滅入ったり、
暗闇に落ちて、うつっぽくなるケースも
少なくありません…

• •

その時どうすればよいか、
ある作曲家が交響曲で表現しました。
本人がひどいうつを体験して、
自殺を考えたこともありました。
彼だけではなく、当時の暗い時代を生きていた人々は
みな落ち込んでいたそうです。
その答えは：元気を出して、喜びを増やすこと。
この洞察が、彼の一番有名な作品になりました。
日本でも大人気の「第九」の話です。
作曲家の名はBeethoven(正発音:ベートホーフェン)。

今回初めて、「第九」の演奏が、
映像(動画)とともに楽しめます。

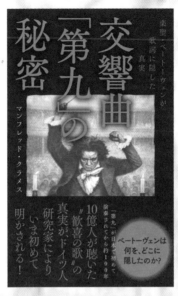

↑M. クラメスの著書。
これを基に「動画第九」が創られました↓

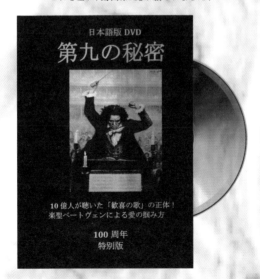

「第九」は
"音楽の神様"といわれる偉大な作曲家、
ベートーヴェンの最後の作品です。
"天使のひらめき"を授かるための
最高傑作であり、
日本でも"聖なる音楽"として
知られています。
その演奏を映像（動画）とともに楽しめます。
涙が出るほど貴方の心を震わせる
保証付き。

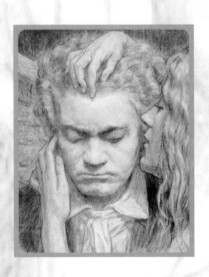

「動画第九」は、M.クラメスが日本で創りました。
「第九」が大好きな日本人に、
曲に隠された真の意味を知らせたいというのが動機です。
作曲家の人物ドキュメンタリーから始まり、
その後、交響曲が美しい映像と
日本語の解説とともに始まります。

全部で100分。
指揮者は有名なHerbert Kegel
演奏は Dresden Philharmonie Orchester
コーラスはBerliner Rundfunkchor & Leipziger
Rundfunkchor
このコンビネーションが成す素晴らしい録音です。

［販売価格］ 2,980円（税込）

> ヒカルランドパーク取扱い商品に関するお問い合わせ等は
> メール：info@hikarulandpark.jp
> URL：http://www.hikaruland.co.jp/
> 03-5225-2671（平日10-17時）

著者のカウンセリング情報

心の病全般、コロナや肺炎の予防、免疫系の強化、様々な症状
の天然薬草での治療、自己自然治療法、お子様のADHD対策
や集中力アップ、不眠、失禁など。
日本に15年滞在したので、日本語堪能です。
現在ドイツ在住のため電話やSkypeもOK。気楽にお問い合わ
せ下さい：Zentai310@gmail.com
※お名前と希望の時間を明記（時差があるため、日本時間の15
時〜 23時までOK。候補日時を2つあげて下さい）

M.クラメスのもう一つの作品をご紹介します
自分らしく生きるためのガイドブック

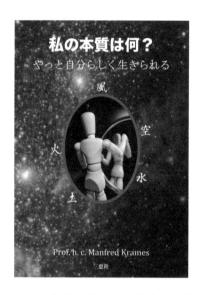

本当に幸せな人たちはみな自分の才能と
それを活かす人生の道すじに気づき、
自分らしい生き方を見つけています。
私たちが生まれつき持っている「五大元素」の割合に、
自分らしさへの「鍵」が隠されています。
その鍵で幸せへの扉をどう開くか、
この本が分かりやすく導きます。

ご購入はAmazonでどうぞ！